Arborvitae

Essential oil

The Generous Tree of Life

By: Stasia Bliss

COPYRIGHT© 2015

First Printing: January 2015

This book and all the books in this series are dedicated to the ever renewed birthing of the Divine Self – for which the gifts of essential oils are continually given.

Table of Contents:

Caution - - Disclaimer - - Personal Health Observation -

This book is not a replacement for therapy, medicines, treatments of any kind. It is merely meant to give a new perspective on the uses of the essential oil mentioned herein.

It is advised that through realizing yourself to be the only One you can change, that when things seem bleak or undesirable, when health or life seems to oppose you, that you instead choose to seek to affect change within yourself rather than look outward for "cures." This book in no way intends to heal or cure you or act as a replacement for medical or psychological treatment, it does intend to lift and inspire you into your own greatness and sovereignty. Proceed at your own risk and free-agency.

"I'm planting a tree to teach me to gather strength from my deepest roots."

— Andrea Koehle Jones, The Wish Trees

Introduction

"*If we will only treat it with the respect in which [the First Peoples] held it, the great west coast cedar will always be with us, to serve with the same regal philanthropy it always has, as a powerfully beautiful asset to our coastal vistas when alive, and as a source of some of the finest materials...*"

~Bill Reid, in his forward to Hilary Stewart's book, Cedar (Douglas & McIntyre, Vancouver, 1984)

Imagine settling within the giant, fragrant trunk of the western red cedar tree, eyes closed, sensing the grandeur of such surroundings. Allow your power of visualization to transport you into the heart of this ancient tree and sense the moist strength of such a gift from Mother Nature. In the heart of what natives call "the tree of life" the essence of its potent oils can be taken in, and there you can be bathed in the rich blessing of that which grew to heal the land and protect itself graciously to live as an immortal – some of the gifts it offers you now.

In the Pacific Northwest region of the United States grows the Western Red Cedar - Thuja Plicata – or Arborvitae – The Tree of Life. It is a rare gift to the planet this majestic tree... some have been around for several thousand years – even as many as 3000-5000 say some.

Standing near one of these trees leaves one in no doubt of its mission here and whether it came equipped to accomplish such a task. It is like a super-hero in the forest, warding off potential invaders with the sweetest of scents and the virtue of anti-destroyer qualities.

If we take a deeper look at how this tree lives and even how it supposedly "dies" we may glean a terrific bulk of insight into how we too may conquer the foes of life and lift ourselves gloriously into the state of immortality and grace.

As the Arborvitae tree stands tall and strong, even in its "fallen" state, so we too may find our greatest gifts in what may appear to be our short-comings.

Let us peer inside the blessed tree of life and how she, and the oils which come from her, may influence our consciousness toward more lofty aspirations and firmer convictions of truth.

Story of Arborvitae –

In the Garden

"The groves were God's first temples."

~William Cullen Bryant~

A Sacred Grove is a forest of trees of spiritual significance to a specific group of people or religion. The Arborvitae tree, also known as the Giant Arborvitae of the Pacific Northwest, has been sacred to the Native American people for as long as it has been known to exist. The story of its creation is attributed to a great man who performed endless generous deeds and after his passing, in the place where he was buried, grew this great tree.

What is beautiful of the story is that traditionally the Native people were not buried prior to this man, but set up in the treetops after they passed. However, it was told to them "Where he is buried, a Cedar tree will grow... And from the boughs, they will brush away illness and sadness."

The Giant Arborvitae literally means *The Tree of Life* as its life is so long, it seems to never die. It continues to give and give of its essence and of the gifts of its form to all that would come to her. This giant tree is not bothered by bugs or insects of any kind, but instead emits a sweet fragrance which allows it to remain pure, strong and blessed.

The Christian story of the Tree of Life could be told with an interesting new twist. Originally, one may understand how after Adam and Eve partook of the Tree of Knowledge that the Tree of Life was then guarded by a cherubim, which many have interpreted to be angels. But if the Giant Arborvitae is seen to be The Tree of Life, full of healing potential and a myriad of gifts for humankind, including the secrets of immortality, then we might consider the Assyrian translation of cherubim or *karabu* – which means "great" and "mighty." In other words, the tree was huge, guarded with mighty properties … as is this majestic tree.

Metaphorically, if one "partakes of the Tree of Knowledge of Good and Evil" they are dropping into the realm of duality, where the polarities of "good" and "bad" as well as "sickness" and "health" exist. With polarity comes both birth and death, pain and pleasure. But, if one learns to take on the attributes of the mighty, great giving tree, the obstacles of duality may be overcome. When this occurs, a person may learn to live in unity consciousness once again, aware of the indwelling divine qualities which perpetuate life continually and protect one from the onslaught of fear, suffering and both inward and outward "attack."

Returning to the garden by utilizing the uplifting and healing properties of Arborvitae essential oil, we are in essence, returning to the sacred grove where the Tree of Life exists within us, and we need not die to it anymore.

Even if we have "fallen," made mistakes or chosen the way of error, we might gain insight and learning from this great tree and see how even after it falls to the ground, it does not lose its virtue, its fragrance or its giving nature. We too may become a people who learns to embrace our follies as the birthing place of our greatest gifts.

Roots God Planted

"Everything on the earth has a purpose, every disease an herb to cure it, and every person a mission. This is the Indian theory of existence."

-Mourning Dove (Salish) 1888-1936

The roots of a tree go largely unseen, yet they are crucial to the development of the tree. Without strong roots, a tree will not grow to its potential, will remain small and will stay disconnected from the rest of the forest, so too, with us.

To be rooted, as a human being, is to be grounded, connected to the Earth on which we live, to be connected to physical life and able to relate to those around us and both give and receive love, compassion and service. If a person is not grounded, they will not be able to reach their fullest potential, they will, in essence, remain small and stay unable to co-create and co-exist with the rest of the human race in harmony and grace.

To be grounded is largely an unseen affair. We do not grow actual roots out of the souls of our feet into the Earth like the trees do. For this reason, it is often easy to mistake that the mere existence of our physical bodies and the ability we have to move about in them equates to being grounded. This is not so.

Have you ever met someone who seemed like they were living in the clouds? The words and concepts escaping their lips simply had no bearing on the world around them, and they seemed unable to connect with you and you with them? We all have been in this state at one time or another, but an individual who is ungrounded, often lives with their minds on things of a spiritual nature and neglects those things which would allow them to exist in the world of form with ease.

Arborvitae essential oil allows one to tap into the roots of existence, to extend energetic grounding rods into the Earth and find feet firmly planted on Terra Firma. It makes one sturdy and trustworthy as the old cedar, able to withstand the winds of mental change and interact with a gracious attitude of blessed giving.

As the oil is used it can stir the lower chakras of the root and the sacral to awaken to their highest expression – that of trust, joy and unique expression. Just as the Giant Western Red Cedar reaches ancient roots into the soils of the Sacred Groves in order to communicate with the forest around it, producing specific oils and resins which would protect it from the very life that might bring it harm, so too can this oil bring interconnection and divine protection to one who would use it with humility.

Physically, Arborvitae essential oil fortifies and strengthens the cells of the body, protecting them from mutation or disease. Spiritually, this oil makes one into the holy temple of the Divine, so the indwelling spirit may reside with loving presence, guarded from the energies and vibrations which would cause one to forget the greatness of their being.

To be rooted in the foundation of truth and trust is essential to the ability for anything to grow tall and strong. Truth comes from an inner alignment with the purpose of Self and trust develops from knowing one's individual purpose is entangled with the Cosmic plan of unfolding life.

Before a tree can grow high into the sky, it must develop its roots. Before a human can reach its greatest potential on this Earth and beyond, they must become grounded in the reality of the place on which they stand. We cannot grow if we deny the grid which translates our life energy into the reality we interact within. We must find a way to plant ourselves deeply into the soil of our lives and develop a foundation from which to rise.

Arborvitae assists one in finding their roots and nourishing them into what they have the purpose of doing – supporting their life.

Healing the Whole Self

"Trees are sanctuaries. Whoever knows how to speak to them, whoever knows how to listen to them, can learn the truth. They do not preach learning and precepts, they preach undeterred by particulars, the ancient law of life."

~ Hermann Hesse ~

Breathing in the deep, rich fragrance of the Arborvitae, it becomes clear there is so much more going on than simple olfactory pleasure. The Earthen aroma of the Red Cedar draws one to connect with the roots of one's existence, but it doesn't stop there. This oil addresses the entire self as a whole structure and leaves no aspect untouched.

Within the body are various systems, all dependent on specific productions, qualities and states of being. It is said that in the presence of fear and emotional disruption, the organs of the body suffer. Chinese medicine reveals how various organ pairs are organized to deal with specific emotions and each pair takes turns in its work to maintain balance and health in the body. Arborvitae creates a positive atmosphere and vibration within the body which allows the organs and cells to remember their original state and move toward that knowing in health and well-being.

Despite the attempts of modern medicine to isolate systems and parts of the body into separate events and worlds, thinking they can address only one area at the exclusion of the rest, there is simply no escaping the fact that we are one system with a myriad of processes. To imagine that the foot is not somehow connected to the head, or the stomach has no bearing on the eyes is to pretend the blood flow and electrical impulses in the body radiate to isolated areas, walled off from the rest and influencing not the others.

Just as the skin covers the entire body, so too does the consciousness super-impose itself over the entire vessel. What must be healed in the small area must be addressed in the whole.

We are but holographic, fractal micro-realities which must be embraced as the wholeness we are. In order to heal the body, the mind or the emotions, the entire system must be brought into harmony and balance.

Arborvitae is a perfect oil for addressing wholeness. Just as the trunk of this great tree is thick and sturdy, filled with the exact combination of components to allow for a long and vibrant existence, so too can its oils imbue us with such qualities and give us the opportunity to connect with the eternal within us – that which does not die – and start to live from this place.

With roots firmly planted in the reality of our life, we can then begin to develop strength and confidence in the vessels we inhabit as being functional and highly responsive to the world around us and the source-light within us.

As this great tree gathers information from its environment through its roots and uses that knowledge to produce the proper alkaloids and compounds in order to extend its life and prosper, so too can the oil of *The Tree of Life* cause us to develop an inner state conducive to the creation of a truly amazing life where we feel abundant and unstoppable.

Using Arborvitae essential oil along the spinal cord can help one to feel deeply supported and assist in activating the entire energy system in the body and rid one from invading viruses or bacteria which would slow one down or cause aging and disease.

Applying over the abdomen and heart area give strength to the front of the body where one might attempt to wear an energetic shield rather than gather the fortitude from within the spirit. Arborvitae can reconnect one with the power inherent within the soul so that energetic and emotional armor are not needed.

"The power of the red cedar was said to be so strong a person could receive strength by standing with his or her back to the tree."

Branches to the Sky

"Your scented leaves

Smell the air

Of sacred smoke

You calm and care."

~ Robin Smalley- From Child-Friendly Narrative

Once we are rooted, with strong bodies, free of illness or weaknesses of any kind, we are able to reach our minds high into the heavens and consider all things of a spiritual nature.

The most wonderful thing this oil offers a person is the ability to both dig deep within the Earth for roots and grounding as well as giving the wings to fly into the realm of the Divine Mind. Arborvitae supplies such a beautiful essence of total harmony, as it derived from the bark of the tree which comprises all of the years of its life. Trees grow wider the older they are. Rings within the trunk tell of the number of years any tree has seen. In the process of creating the sacred shavings, though a waste product before this oil was captured, now an opportunity to utilize every aspect of the great tree on every level. For once the trunk has gifted its strength to what will be created from it, the "left-overs" still contain perhaps the greatest gift of all – the essential oil.

In this awareness, may an insight be gained. For it is after we have given our all in the world in which we dwell, in service and love to humanity, that we are able to reap the benefits of "what is left" of us. The essence of the spirit seems to come through clearly and most purely from the heart who has so freely given. The essential oil is like the blood of the tree, harvested from the bark chips left from the milling.

When we give our lives in the service of something greater, we often feel sapped and exhausted to the bone, as if nothing is left of us. Ah, but this is when the grace of spirit takes over and shows us that our true strengths lies not in that which is material, but in the ability we then have to reach the heights of ecstasy in surrender to spirit. Note how this is only possible *after* the giving of all that we have.

The branches of our existence grow into the heavens through much discipline on our part, to give, and sacrifice lovingly in the service of others. You could say the branches are the reward for a trunk well grown. As we nourish the physical and connect through our roots to the community in which we are placed, we are gifted antennas which reach into the realm of spirit, where gifts may be given us in the form of fruits... those things which bless not only us, but those around us even more.

Arborvitae strengthens our roots, nourishes our bodies and inspires our branches into the heavens. It is the gift of the Divine in a time when so much confusion has reigned upon the Earth. It is only now that the forests give their secrets. The holy groves begin to speak and tell the stories of immortality in the way they live and breathe and have their existence.

"...only the trees, only the trees....like a key they see beyond the mystery, waiting endlessly...ever holding me, like I hold the sky."

~Stasia Bliss original poem *Sky*

All Other Reasons Why

"These are the secrets of the trees."

-Jami Seiber – Cellist

The Arborvitae tree is one of the closest physical representation on Earth that we have to what it looks like to be immortal. It stands tall and gives continually, even after it has turned horizontal, still, nothing may destroy it, save ax and mill – and even then, its essence continues on in a myriad of glorious forms.

As each one of us decide to live more conscious, aware lives where we take note of the way we are grounded, the stature of our bodies and allow for connection with the Divine, we become more akin to this great tree. The Giant Arborvitae - in the form of therapeutic grade essential oils – can imbue us with the proper vibration we need to align with the energy of The

Tree of Life, to become at one with the Source of creation.

Through regular use of this oil, the cells of the body can learn to create themselves anew in the likeness of health, vitality and truth. We need not suffer the mutations of physical life where we tend toward carrying the sorrow and pain of the day to day within us. No. Instead, we may learn to keep our burden light, to drop away that which no longer serves as we are lifted up in the essence of the great trees, the sacred groves of the world – within our own beings.

Arborvitae essential oil is truly a gift of the Divine, sourced from the purest region held in pristine recognition of the sacred value of its life and essence. Since there is currently only one source for this oil, one who uses it can be certain of its purity and high intention, to serve humanity as it has served from the beginning of its life.

How to Best Use Arborvitae

Essential oil

In the Bath -

In the bathtub one may connect with the element of water and the substance which makes up the largest percentage of the physical body. Using Arborvitae in the bath can help to sooth the emotional state and bring healing vibrations to the entire body system as the skin takes in this pure essence through the medium of water.

By taking time to meditate in the bath on the strength of the Arborvitae one may activate, more fully, that inherent strength within and emerge feeling lighter and more connected.

Breathe it in —

Diffusing this tree oil into the atmosphere can make one feel like they are walking through the great forests of the Pacific Northwest. The smell permeates the environment and assists one in lifting their minds to a higher plane of reality in order to dwell on thoughts of a higher nature.

If emotions are troubled or mental states are in too much constant flux, Arborvitae can help bring harmony and balance into a person. This oil can also assist one in finding proper grounding, building a foundation of trust in life and stepping forward to create the reality they desire – in alignment with their highest truth.

This oil can also greatly assist the respiratory system in more fluid movement and deeper breathing with ease. In this way, it also helps one to become more finely attuned to spirit and the "breath of the divine" in how it communicates to an individual. It may increase ones capacity to breathe deeper and practice awareness of body "prana" – or life-force in the breath.

Arborvitae is particularly suited for yoga practitioners or those working with the breath and body movement. It would be ideal to infuse a yoga room with the scent of this tree in order to inspire body-connectivity along with soul realization and community at-one-ment.

Topically –

Arborvitae applied directly to the skin can bring instant change to a situation or sensation. It can help to open one up and remove blocks of stubbornness or superiority. Just as the great red cedar knows that it shares the forest with other trees and therefore must remain in harmony with them, Arborvitae assists a person in recognizing ones role in life as well as the purpose of others on their path.

A sensitive person may feel sensitive to power of Arborvitae on the skin, though its oil is gentle enough to be applied neat, in most cases.

Souls of the Feet – applied to the feet, this oil can assist one in grounding to the Earth and feeling the supportive energies available to all from the core of the great Mama. If one is feeling stuck, unable to move, Arborvitae can help mobilize one into action by noticing the opportunities presenting themselves in day-to-day life.

Top of the Head – applied to the crown, Arborvitae can connect one to the realm of the Divine more purely. It has the potential to sweep away worries and allow one a more clear communication of inspiration and insight. It may relieve one of mental pressures and the tendency to dwell on the inharmonious. The third eye can be gently stimulated into action and dream-states can be more fully recollected. This oil is ideal for meditation and harmonizing both hemispheres of the brain, supporting Alpha rhythms and peace.

Heart – Over the heart center, Arborvitae helps to gently open a closed heart and remove blocks that have kept one from connecting to others emotionally. It can assist one in developing unconditional love and the ability to self-heal by tuning one into the inherent energies of wholeness within.

Naval – Over the belly, Arborvitae assist in digestion by helping one with the capacity to take in life anew, repelling the negative or "harmful" factors and assimilating the beneficial – which can result in a more fine-tuned digestive system. It may also help activate one's personal power which comes from feeling fully grounded and in contact with the Divine.

Divine Child of the Universe, anoint thyself with oils for thine own remembrance, for Ye are Gods!

Arborvitae shows one the way, within the vessel of the body, to immortality, by uplifting the soul into resonance with ones truest nature. It can help to extend the life by canceling out feelings of negativity and doubt, which suppress the light of the spirit and block authenticity.

Resources:

doTERRA essential oils – doterrauniversity.com

http://www.greatdreams.com/native/spirit-keepers.htm

Sourcing video - http://vimeo.com/108507165

VandusenBloedelBotanicalGarden: http://vandusengarden.org/explore/vandusen-botanical-garden/plant-collections/tree-month/western-redcedar

To buy this oil visit: www.mydoterra.com/blissinthehouse

www.ingramcontent.com/pod-product-compliance
Lightning Source LLC
Chambersburg PA
CBHW061929280526
45787CB00004B/1545